HIGH-PROTEIN VEGETARIAN DIET PLAN COOK BOOK

A Comprehensive Plan for a High-Protein Vegetarian Diet and Its Advantages for Your Health

REX LEWIS

Table of Contents

Introduction

The High-Protein Vegetarian Diet Emphasizes Fulfilling Increased Protein Requirements Mostly Through Plant-Based Sources And Excludes Meat And Animal Products. High-Protein Diets Focus On The Abundant Protein Content In Different Plant Sources, Challenging The Common Belief That They Are Only Associated With Animal Protein Consumption. Individuals Adopting A High-Protein Vegetarian Diet Attempt To Optimize Protein Consumption For Various Health Advantages By Including A Variety Of Plant-Based Foods Such Legumes, Tofu, Tempeh, Nuts, Seeds, And Grains.

People Often Choose This Diet For A Variety Of Reasons, Such As Health And Fitness Objectives, Ethical Concerns About Animal Cruelty, And Environmental Sustainability Issues. Plant-Based Proteins Support Muscle Maintenance And Growth While Providing Important Minerals, Fiber, And Phytochemicals That Enhance Overall Health.

The High-Protein Vegetarian Diet Integrates Nutritional Research, Ethical Ideals, And Environmental Awareness, Emphasizing A Comprehensive Approach To Health That Considers Societal And Ecological Effects. As People Hunt For Diets That Match Their Values And Health Goals,

The High-Protein Vegetarian Diet Is A Suitable Choice For Those Aiming To Increase Their Protein Intake While Following A Plant-Based Lifestyle.

CHAPTER ONE
Comprehending Protein In A Vegetarian Diet

Comprehending The Role Of Protein In A Vegetarian Diet Is Essential To Ensure That Those Adhering To Plant-Based Eating Habits Receive Sufficient Nourishment For Optimal Health. Key Aspects To Consider Are:

• Protein Requirements Depend On Parameters Like Age, Sex, And Activity Level, And Are Determined By The Recommended Dietary Allowance (RDA). Adults Are Advised To Consume Approximately 0.8 Grams Of Protein Per Kilogram Of Body Weight On Average. Nevertheless, Certain Individuals, Such As Sportsmen Or

That Pursuing Muscle Growth, May Necessitate Increased Quantities.

- **Plant-Based Protein Sources:** Vegetarians Can Acquire Protein From Legumes, Tofu, Tempeh, Edamame, Nuts, Seeds, Whole Grains Including Quinoa, Brown Rice, Oats, And Plant-Based Protein Supplements.

- **Protein Complementation:** Some Plant Proteins May Be Deficient In Some Necessary Amino Acids, Unlike Animal Proteins. By Combining Several Plant-Based Protein Sources, Individuals Can Guarantee They Receive A Comprehensive Amino Acid Profile. Combining Beans With Rice Or Whole-Grain Bread With Nut Butter Can Produce Complementing Proteins.

• **Quantity And Distribution:** Distributing Protein Intake Evenly Throughout The Day Enhances Muscle Protein Synthesis. Adding Protein To Every Meal And Snack Can Help Achieve A More Stable And Prolonged Release Of Amino Acids.

• Plant-Based Proteins May Have Poorer Digestion And Absorption Rates Than Animal Proteins. Properly Cooking And Preparing Plant-Based Foods, Together With Incorporating Sources High In Essential Amino Acids, Can Improve Protein Absorption.

• **Fortified Meals:** Certain Plant-Based Meals Are Enriched With Extra Protein, Like Specific Plant-Based Milk Substitutes And Goods Fortified With

Protein. Examining Food Labels Might Assist In Recognizing Fortified Choices.

• Prioritizing Nutrient-Dense Plant-Based Foods Guarantees Individuals Receive Protein Along With Vital Vitamins, Minerals, Fiber, And Antioxidants Crucial For Overall Well-Being.

• **Variety And Balance:** A Broad And Well-Balanced Diet Is Essential For Fulfilling All Nutritional Requirements. Incorporating A Diverse Range Of Vegetables, Fruits, Whole Grains, And Plant-Based Proteins Is Essential For Achieving A Well-Rounded Nutrient Profile.

• Supplementation May Be Opted For By Individuals To Fulfill Certain Protein Needs By Incorporating Plant-Based Protein Powders Or Other Supplements Into Their Diet. Seeking Advice From A Healthcare Expert Or Dietitian Can Help Determine Suitable Supplementation.

• Proper Hydration Is Crucial For Optimum Protein Metabolism And Overall Well-Being. Water Is Essential For Several Physiological Functions, Such As Digestion And Nutrition Absorption.

Comprehending These Elements Of Protein In A Vegetarian Diet Enables Individuals To Make Knowledgeable Dietary Decisions, Promoting Their

Health And Well-Being While Following A Plant-Based Lifestyle. Seeking Advice From A Licensed Dietitian Can Offer Tailored Recommendations According To Personal Dietary Choices, Health Objectives, And Nutritional Requirements.

Advantages of a High-Protein Vegetarian Diet

A High-Protein Vegetarian Diet Can Give Numerous Health Advantages If Individuals Make Careful And Well-Rounded Dietary Selections. Here Are Some Possible Benefits:

• High-Protein Diets, Including Vegetarian Options, Can Aid With Weight Management. Protein Can

Enhance Sensations Of Fullness And Satiety, Leading To A Decrease In Total Calorie Consumption And Supporting Weight Reduction Or Weight Maintenance.

• Protein Is Crucial For The Maintenance And Growth Of Muscles. Vegetarians Can Get Sufficient Protein From Plant-Based Sources Such Beans, Tofu, Tempeh, Seitan, And Plant-Based Protein Supplements.

• A Well-Designed High-Protein Vegetarian Diet Can Have A High Nutritional Density, Containing Vital Nutrients Such As Fiber, Vitamins, And Minerals. Consuming A Diverse Range Of Plant-Based Foods Provides A Wide

Array Of Nutrients, Which Enhances Overall Health.

• Plant-Based Proteins Often Contain Less Saturated Fat Than Animal-Based Proteins, Promoting Heart Health. Consuming A Diet Rich In Plant Proteins Can Improve Heart Health By Lowering Cholesterol Levels And Blood Pressure.

• **Enhanced Blood Sugar Regulation:** Vegetarian Diets High In Protein, Particularly Those With A Low Glycemic Index, Can Assist In Maintaining Stable Blood Sugar Levels. This Could Be Advantageous For Persons With Diabetes Or Those Susceptible To Acquiring Diabetes.

- Plant-Based Protein Sources Including Beans, Lentils, And Whole Grains Are High In Fiber, Which Benefits Digestive Health. Sufficient Fiber Consumption Aids In Maintaining Digestive Health By Reducing Constipation And Fostering A Healthy Gut Micro Biota.

- Some Research Indicates That Following A High-Protein Vegetarian Diet Could Lower The Likelihood Of Developing Specific Chronic Diseases Such As Cardiovascular Disease And Some Types Of Malignancies.

- Plant-Based Proteins Are Typically More Environmentally Sustainable Than Animal-Based Proteins. Opting For A High-Protein Vegetarian Diet

Can Help Increase Sustainability By Decreasing The Environmental Impact Linked To Animal Agriculture.

• Plant-Based Proteins Are Potentially Less Taxing On The Kidneys Than Large Quantities Of Animal Protein, Promoting Kidney Health. This Is Particularly Important For Persons With Kidney Problems Or Those Susceptible To Kidney Disease.

• Ethical And Animal Welfare Considerations: Opting For A Vegetarian Diet Is In Line With Ethical And Animal Welfare Concerns. Many Individuals Choose To Follow A Vegetarian Lifestyle Due To Concerns About Animal Welfare And Environmental Sustainability.

The Key To Maintaining A Balanced High-Protein Vegetarian Diet Is To Prioritize Diversity, Balance, And Adequate Planning To Guarantee The Intake Of All Vital Elements. Seeking Guidance From A Healthcare Expert Or A Certified Dietitian Can Assist In Developing A Customized Nutrition Plan Tailored To Individual Requirements And Objectives.

CHAPTER TWO
Designing Your High-Protein Vegetarian Diet

To Design A High-Protein Vegetarian Diet Effectively, Individuals Must Carefully Examine Their Nutritional Requirements And Aim For A Wide And Balanced Selection Of Plant-Based Foods. Here Is A Strategy For Creating A High-Protein Vegetarian Diet.

1. Calculate Protein Requirements:

• Calculate Your Specific Protein Requirements By Considering Criteria Including Age, Gender, Weight, Physical Activity, And Health Objectives. The Recommended Dietary Allowance (RDA) Serves As A General Guideline, But, Certain Individuals

Such As Athletes May Require Higher Protein Intake.

2. Opt For A Range Of Plant-Based Protein Sources In Your Diet. Examples Include Of Legumes, Tofu, Tempeh, Edamame, Almonds, Seeds, Whole Grains, And Plant-Based Protein Supplements.

3. Maintain A Balanced Distribution Of Macronutrients By Including Carbs And Healthy Fats In Addition To Proteins. A Well-Rounded Diet Includes Whole Grains, Fruits, Vegetables, And Plant-Based Fats Such As Avocado, Nuts, And Seeds.

4. Enhance Amino Acid Profile:

• Blend Different Plant-Based Protein Sources To Guarantee A Comprehensive Array Of Important Amino Acids. Examples Include Combining Beans With Rice Or Quinoa, Or Matching Whole-Grain Bread With Nut Butter.

5. Meal Planning: Plan Meals That Incorporate A Protein Source Such Beans, Lentils, Tofu, Or Tempeh. Include A Diverse Selection Of Vibrant Vegetables, Complete Grains, And Nutritious Fats To Make Fulfilling And Nourishing Meals.

6. Consume A Protein Source With Every Meal And Snack To Promote

Muscle Maintenance And Feelings Of Fullness. Options Include Plant-Based Yogurt, Almonds, A Protein-Rich Smoothie, Or A Plant-Based Protein Snack.

7. Incorporate Fortified Plant-Based Foods, Like Certain Plant-Based Milk Replacements, To Guarantee Sufficient Consumption Of Nutrients Such As Vitamin B12 And Calcium.

8. Hydration: Maintain Proper Hydration. Water Is Essential For Maintaining Good Health And Aids In Digestion And The Absorption Of Nutrients, Particularly Protein Metabolism.

9. Monitor Portion Amounts: Be Attentive To Portion Amounts To Prevent Overeating. Protein Is Crucial, But It Is Equally Necessary To Ensure A Balance With Other Nutrients.

10. Experiment With Meals:

• Try Out Different Vegetarian Meals To Maintain A Diverse And Satisfying Diet. There Are Numerous Innovative Methods To Create Plant-Based Meals That Are Rich In Protein And Flavor.

11. Seek Consultation From A Licensed Dietitian For Individualized Recommendations On Fulfilling Dietary Needs And Particular Health Goals.

12. Consider Additional Vital Minerals Including Iron, Calcium, Zinc, Vitamin D, And Omega-3 Fatty Acids. Incorporate A Diverse Selection Of Foods To Guarantee A Balanced Nutrient Composition.

13. Be Attentive To Your Body:

• Notice Signals Of Hunger And Satiety. Modify Your Food According To Your Energy Levels, Performance, And General Well-Being.

By Applying These Concepts, People Can Develop A High-Protein Vegetarian Diet That Is Both Nutritionally Balanced And Pleasant, As Well As Sustainable In The Long Run.

Essential Nutrients in a Vegetarian Diet

A Balanced Vegetarian Diet Can Supply All The Vital Elements Needed For Optimal Health. Although Nutrient Requirements Differ Across Individuals, Here Are Essential Nutrients To Focus On In A Vegetarian Diet:

• Protein Sources Include Legumes (Beans, Lentils, and Chickpeas), Tofu, Tempeh, Edamame, Almonds, Seeds, And Whole Grains.

• Consider Using Protein Complementation To Achieve A Comprehensive Amino Acid Profile.

- Iron Sources Include Dark Leafy Greens (Such As Spinach And Kale), Legumes, Fortified Cereals, Whole Grains, Nuts, And Seeds.

Improve Iron Absorption By Eating Foods High In Vitamin C With Foods High In Iron.

- Calcium Sources Include Fortified Plant-Based Milk (Soy, Almond, Oat), Tofu, Leafy Greens (Collard Greens, Bok Choy), Almonds, And Sesame Seeds.

Strive For Sufficient Calcium Consumption, Particularly If Dairy Is Being Avoided.

- Vitamin B12 Sources Include Fortified Foods Such As Plant-Based

Milk, Cereals, And Nutritional Yeast, As Well As B12 Pills.

Consider Supplementing With B12 Since It Is Mostly Present In Animal Food.

•   Omega-3 Fatty Acids Can Be Acquired Via Flaxseeds, Chia Seeds, Walnuts, Hemp Seeds, And Algae-Based Supplements.

• Incorporate Plant-Based Sources Or Contemplate   Omega-3 Supplementation.

• Zinc Sources Include Legumes, Nuts, Seeds, And Whole Grains.

• Ensure Adequate Zinc Consumption, As Plant-Based Sources May Have Reduced Bioavailability.

• Vitamin D Sources Include Sun Exposure, Fortified Plant-Based Milk, And Vitamin D2/D3 Pills.

Monitor Vitamin D Levels, Particularly In Cases Of Reduced Sun Exposure.

• Iodine Sources Include Iodized Salt, Seaweed, And Iodine Supplements If Necessary.

Ensure Enough Iodine Consumption, As Many Plant-Based Diets May Lack Sufficient Iodine.

• Fiber Sources Include Fruits, Vegetables, Whole Grains, And Legumes.

Plant-Based Diets Typically Contain Abundant Fiber, Which Supports Digestive Health.

• Magnesium Sources Include Nuts, Seeds, Whole Grains, Leafy Greens, And Legumes.

Consume Sufficient Magnesium To Support Multiple Physiological Activities.

• Vitamin A Sources Include Beta-Carotene-Rich Foods Such As Carrots, Sweet Potatoes, And Spinach, As Well As Fruits.

Eat A Diverse Selection Of Colorful Fruits And Vegetables To Obtain Vitamin A Precursors.

• Vitamin E Sources Include Nuts, Seeds, Spinach, Broccoli, And Plant Oils.

Include Vitamin E Sources For Antioxidant Advantages.

• Folate, Also Known As Vitamin B9, Can Be Found In Leafy Greens, Lentils, And Fortified Cereals.

Ensure An Adequate Intake Of Folate, Particularly For Women Of Reproductive Age.

• Potassium Sources Include Bananas, Potatoes, Sweet Potatoes, Oranges, Tomatoes, And Beans.

Eat Meals High In Potassium To Promote Heart And Muscle Health.

• Phosphorus Sources Include Nuts, Seeds, Whole Grains, Legumes, And Tofu.

Ensure A Proper Equilibrium Between Phosphorus And Calcium Consumption.

Consuming A Diverse Range Of Plant-Based Foods And Utilizing Supplements When Needed Helps Vegetarians Fulfill Their Nutritional Requirements. Seeking Advice From A Licensed Dietician Can Offer Tailored Recommendations According To Specific Health Objectives, Tastes, And Possible Nutritional Deficiencies.

CHAPTER THREE
Protein-Rich Foods for Vegetarians

Vegetarians Can Select From A Diverse Range Of Plant-Based Foods High In Protein To Fulfill Their Nutritional Requirements. Below Are Some High-Quality Protein Sources Suitable For Persons Adhering To A Vegetarian Diet:

1. Legumes: Lentils - Chickpeas - Black Beans - Kidney Beans - Peas

2. Tofu And Tempeh: - Tofu Comes In Varieties Such As Silken, Firm, And Extra Firm. - Tempeh Is A Fermented Soybean Food.

3. Edamame: Young, Green Soybeans

4. Quinoa Is A Complete Protein Grain.

5. Whole Grains Include Brown Rice, Barley, Farro, Bulgur, And Oats.

6. Nuts And Seeds: Almonds - Walnuts - Peanuts - Chia Seeds - Flaxseeds - Hemp Seeds - Sunflower Seeds - Pumpkin Seeds

7. Seitan Is A Protein Derived From Wheat Gluten.

8. Dairy Substitutes: Plant-Based Greek Yogurt - Plant-Based Milk Options (Soy, Almond, Oat) - Non-Dairy Cheese Alternatives

9. Eggs Are Suitable For Ovo Vegetarians.

10. Plant-Based Protein Powders Include Pea, Rice, Hemp, And Soy Protein.

11. Nutritional Yeast Is Enriched With Protein And Vitamin B12.

12. Legume-Based Pastas Include Chickpea Pasta And Lentil Pasta.

13. Vegetarian Meat Substitutes Include Veggie Burgers, Veggie Sausages, And Plant-Based Deli Slices.

14. Spirulina And Chlorella Are Blue-Green Algae With High Protein Content.

15. Soy Products: Soybeans, Soy Milk, Soy Nuts

By Incorporating A Diverse Selection Of Protein-Rich Foods In Their Meals And Snacks, Vegetarians Can Guarantee They Receive A Comprehensive Blend Of Amino Acids And Critical Nutrients. Integrating Various Protein Sources Into Your Daily Meals Can Help Maintain A Well-Rounded And Healthy Diet. Seeking Advice From A Licensed Dietitian Can Offer Tailored Recommendations According To Personal Dietary Choices, Health Objectives, And Nutritional Requirements.

High-Protein Vegetarian Recipes.

Certainly! Here Are Three Vegetarian Meals High In Protein, Which Are Both Tasty And Rich In Plant-Based Protein.

1. Quinoa and Black Bean Bowl:

Ingredients:

• 1 Cup Cooked Quinoa

• 1 Can Drained And Rinsed Black Beans

• 1 Cup Corn Kernels (Fresh Or Frozen)

• 1 Cup Halved Cherry Tomatoes

• 1 Diced Avocado

• 1/4 Cup Finely Chopped Red Onion

• Chopped Fresh Cilantro

- Lime Wedges

- Salt And Pepper To Taste

Directions:

1. Mix Cooked Quinoa, Black Beans, Corn, Cherry Tomatoes, Avocado, And Red Onion In A Large Bowl.

2. Combine Thoroughly And Season With Salt And Pepper.

Garnish With Chopped Cilantro And Serve With Lime Wedges To Enhance The Flavor.

2. Lentil and Vegetable Stir-Fry:

Ingredients:

- 1 Cup Cooked Green Or Brown Lentils

- 2 Cups Broccoli Florets

- 1 Sliced Red Bell Pepper

- 1 Julienned Carrot

- 1 Sliced Zucchini

- 3 Minced Cloves of Garlic

- 1 Tablespoon Grated Ginger

- 1/4 Cup Soy Sauce

- 2 Tbsp Sesame Oil

- Chopped Green Onions For Garnish

- Sesame Seeds For Garnish

Directions:

1. Heat Sesame Oil in a Large Wok or Skillet over Medium-High Heat.

2. Sauté Garlic And Ginger For 1-2 Minutes Until Aromatic.

3. Include Broccoli, Bell Pepper, Carrot, And Zucchini. Sauté For 5-7 Minutes Until Vegetables Are Al Dente.

4. Combine Cooked Lentils With Soy Sauce, Whisk Well, And Heat.

5. Garnish With Diced Scallions And Sesame Seeds Prior To Serving.

3. Curry Made With Chickpeas And Spinach:

Ingredients:

- 2 Cans Chickpeas, Drained And Rinsed

- 1 Large Onion, Finely Chopped

- 3 Cloves Garlic, Minced

- 1 Tablespoon Ginger, Grated

- 1 Can Diced Tomatoes

- 1 Can Coconut Milk

- 3 Cups Fresh Spinach

- 2 Tablespoons Curry Powder

- 1 Teaspoon Turmeric

- 1 Teaspoon Cumin

- Salt And Pepper To Taste

- Cooked Brown Rice or Quinoa for Serving

Directions:

1. In a Large Pan, Cook Onions, Garlic, and Ginger Until They Are Softened.
2. Combine Curry Powder, Turmeric, And Cumin. Mix Thoroughly.
3. Add Diced Tomatoes And Coconut Milk. Cook Over Low Heat For 5 Minutes.
4. Incorporate Chickpeas And Simmer For An Extra 10-15 Minutes.
5. Add Fresh Spinach And Stir Until It Wilts. Season With Salt And Pepper.
6. Serve On Top Of Cooked Brown Rice Or Quinoa.

Feel At Liberty To Adapt These Recipes To Suit Your Tastes And Dietary Requirements. They Offer A Significant Protein Content And A Pleasurable Culinary Experience For Anyone Adhering To A Vegetarian Diet.

Meal Preparation Strategies

Meal Planning Is A Beneficial Method For Saving Time, Adhering To A Healthy Diet, And Alleviating Stress Throughout The Week. Here Are Some Strategies To Enhance The Efficiency And Enjoyment Of Your Meal Preparation Sessions:

Plan:

- Develop A Weekly Menu By Planning Meals For Breakfast, Lunch, Dinner, And Snacks.

- Maintain Nutritional Balance By Incorporating Protein, Carbs, Healthy Fats, And A Variety Of Veggies In Your Meals.

- Batch Cooking: Designate One Or Two Days Weekly To Prepare A Large Quantity Of Items That May Be Utilized In Various Meals.

- Begin with Simple Recipes That Involve Few Materials And Minimum Preparation.

Implementation:

• Utilize A Range Of Containers Of Various Sizes To Keep Meals And Snacks Effectively. Select Containers That Are Both Microwave And Dishwasher-Safe.

• Prepare Protein In Huge Quantities By Cooking Significant Amounts Of Protein Sources Such As Beans, Lentils, And Tofu, Then Divide Them Into Portions For Various Meals.

• Prepare Vegetables Ahead Of Time By Washing, Chopping, And Storing Them For Convenient Use When Preparing Meals. Certain Vegetables Can Be Diced And Preserved In The Freezer.

• Pre-Cook Grains Such As Quinoa, Brown Rice, Or Farro To Serve As A Foundation For Several Meals During The Week.

• Create Dressings, Sauces, Or Marinades Ahead Of Time For Convenient Flavor Enhancements.

• Use Slow Cookers Or Instant Pots To Effortlessly Cook Big Amounts Of Food.

Storage:

• Label Your Containers With The Date Of Preparation To Monitor Freshness.

• Freeze Individual Portions Of Soups, Stews, Or Casseroles To Extend Their Shelf Life.

- Utilize Stackable Containers To Optimize Space In Your Refrigerator Or Freezer.

Diversity:

- Rotate Recipes Weekly To Maintain Variety And Interest.

- Prepare Nutritious Snacks Such As Sliced Fruits, Vegetables, And Hummus For Convenient Snacking.

Efficiency Tips:

- Multi-Task By Cooking Various Components At The Same Time To Be More Time-Efficient.

- Practice Good Hygiene By Washing Dishes And Tidying Up After Each Step To Prevent A Large Mess Later On.

• Prepare Breakfast In Advance By Prepping Overnight Oats, Chia Seed Pudding, Or Smoothie Ingredients The Night Before For A Convenient Morning Meal.

Remain Orderly:

• Conduct Regular Inventory Checks Of Your Pantry And Refrigerator To Ensure Timely Usage Of Items Before They Expire.

• Establish A Certain Day For Consuming Leftovers To Minimize Food Wastage.

• Maintain A Well-Stocked Pantry With Essential Items Such As Canned Beans, Tomatoes, Spices, And Grains For Convenient Meal Preparation.

Meal Planning Is Adaptable And Can Be Customized According To Your Tastes And Timetable. Explore Many Tactics Till You Discover The Most Effective One For You.

Selecting High-Quality Supplements

It Is Essential To Select High-Quality Supplements To Guarantee That You Are Receiving Safe And Efficient Items That Fulfill Your Nutritional Requirements. Here Are Some Guidelines To Assist You In Choosing Premium Supplements:

• Seek Supplements That Have Undergone Independent Testing By Third-Party Organizations Like NSF, Informed-Choice, Or USP. This

Guarantees That The Product Has Been Confirmed For Quality And Effectiveness.

• **Quality Certifications:** - Look For Quality Certifications On The Supplement Label, Including GMP (Good Manufacturing Practices), Which Signifies That The Product Is Manufactured In Accordance With Industry Norms.

• **Bioavailability:** Take Into Account The Nutritional Form Present In The Supplement. Certain Kinds Are More Readily Assimilated By The Body Than Others. Opt For Vitamin D3 Instead Of D2 And Methylcobalamin Over Cyanocobalamin For Vitamin B12.

• Choose Supplements With Few Chemicals, Fillers, And Artificial Colors. Examine The Ingredient List To Verify The Absence Of Any Superfluous Or Potentially Hazardous Chemicals.

• Verify Allergy Information, Particularly If You Have Sensitivities Or Allergies. Certain Supplements May Include Typical Allergies Such As Gluten, Soy, Or Dairy.

• Opt For Items With Transparent Labeling That Clearly Indicates The Quantity Of Each Nutrient Per Serving. Avoid Using Proprietary Mixes Since They May Not Provide Information On The Specific Amounts Of Various Ingredients.

• Investigate The Brand By Seeking For Respectable And Well-Established Brands. Investigate The Company's Reputation, Manufacturing Procedures, And Dedication To Quality.

• Utilize Supplements From Companies That Specialize In The Precise Type Of Supplement Required. A Company That Specializes In Fish Oil May Offer A Superior Omega-3 Supplement Compared To A General Supplement Manufacturer.

• Verify The Presence Of A Clearly Marked Expiration Date On The Supplement. Expired Vitamins May Be Less Effective.

• Consult Healthcare Professionals, Such As A Doctor Or Certified Nutritionist, Before Initiating Any New Supplement Program. They Can Offer Customized Guidance According To Your Health Condition And Dietary Requirements.

• Avoid Supplements That Make Unrealistic Or Excessive Claims. Supplements Should Enhance A Nutritious Diet, Not Substitute For It Or Guarantee Extraordinary Outcomes.

• Whole Food Supplements, Sourced From Actual Food, May Offer A More Complete Nutrient Profile Than Synthetic Alternatives.

• Evaluate The Reputation Of The Supplement By Checking Internet Reviews And Seeking Suggestions From Reliable Sources To Understand The Experiences Of Other Customers.

Keep In Mind That Supplements Are Meant To Complement, Not Substitute, A Well-Rounded Diet. Strive To Get Nutrition From Entire Foods Whenever You Can. When Supplementing, Choose Wisely According To Your Specific Health Objectives And Requirements.

CHAPTER FOUR
Plant-Based Protein Digestibility

Plant-Based Protein Digestibility Can Fluctuate Depending On The Protein Source, Processing Techniques, And Individual Variations In Digestive Systems. Although Plant Proteins May Have Slightly Lower Digestibility Than Animal Proteins, Consuming A Diverse Range Of Plant-Based Protein Sources And Utilizing Specific Preparation Techniques Might Improve Their Bioavailability. Here Are Some Essential Aspects Concerning The Digestion Of Plant-Derived Proteins:

• Plant Proteins May Lack Certain Critical Amino Acids Unlike Animal Proteins. By Combining Various Plant

Protein Sources Like Beans With Rice Or Lentils With Whole Grains, People Can Construct Complete Protein Profiles, Which Improve Overall Amino Acid Absorption.

• Cooking And Processing Techniques Can Impact The Digestion Of Plant Proteins. Soaking And Sprouting Legumes And Grains Can Decrease Anti-Nutrients, Therefore Enhancing The Digestibility Of Proteins. Cooking Helps To Break Down Intricate Protein Structures, Which Assists With Digestion.

• Fermentation Of Plant-Based Meals Like Tempeh And Miso Enhances Digestibility And Boosts Nutritional Bioavailability, Particularly Proteins.

Protein Isolates And Concentrates, Obtained From Plants, Are Highly Purified Types Of Protein That Often Include Higher Protein Levels And Better Digestibility Than Entire Meals. Examples Include Of Pea Protein Isolate Or Soy Protein Concentrate.

• Enzyme Supplements Can Help Folks Digest Plant-Based Proteins More Effectively. Beano Contains Enzymes That Aid In The Digestion Of Specific Complex Carbohydrates Present In Beans And Other Legumes.

• There Is Individual Variability In Digestive Tolerance. Individuals May Encounter Gas Or Bloating When First Increasing Their Consumption Of Some Plant-Based Proteins. Slowly

Incorporating These Meals And Observing The Body's Reactions Can Aid In Pinpointing Any Sensitivities.

• Some Plant-Based Protein Sources Have Great Digestibility. Examples Include Of Tofu and Tempeh (Soy Products), Quinoa, Pea Protein, Lentils, Edamame, And Spirulina.

• A Balanced Diet Consisting Of A Diverse Range Of Plant-Based Protein Sources, Fiber, Vitamins, And Minerals Promotes Optimal Digestive Health.

• **Hydration:** Proper Hydration Is Crucial For Healthy Digestion, Which Includes The Breakdown And Absorption Of Proteins.

Although Some Plant Proteins May Be Less Digestible Than Some Animal Proteins, It Is Feasible To Fulfill Protein Requirements With A Well Designed And Diverse Plant-Based Diet. Those With Particular Concerns Or Digestive Problems Should Seek Advice From A Healthcare Professional Or Certified Dietitian For Tailored Guidance.

Vegan Fitness and Exercise

Vegetarians, Just Like Everyone Else, Can Gain Advantages From A Comprehensive Fitness And Exercise Regimen. Exercise Is Crucial For Maintaining Good Health And Works Well With A Plant-Based Diet To Improve Cardiovascular Health,

Physical Strength, Flexibility, And Mental Well-Being. Here Are Some Suggestions And Tips For Integrating Fitness Into A Vegetarian Lifestyle:

1. Select A Diverse Range Of Workouts Including Cardiovascular Activities (Such As Running, Cycling, Or Swimming), Strength Training (With Weights Or Resistance Bands), And Flexibility Exercises (Like Yoga Or Stretching).

2. Establish Realistic Fitness Goals That Are In Line With Your Overall Health Objectives. Possible Goals May Involve Weight Control, Muscle Development, Improved Flexibility, Or Increased Stamina.

3. Strength Training: Incorporate Strength Training Activities To Develop And Sustain Muscular Mass. Beans, Lentils, Tofu, And Plant-Based Protein Supplements Can Aid In Muscle Rehabilitation And Growth As They Are Rich Sources Of Plant-Based Protein.

4. Cardiovascular Exercise:

• Participate In Aerobic Exercises To Promote Heart Health. Running, Cycling, Swimming, And Dancing Are Excellent Choices. An Adequately Balanced Vegetarian Diet Provide The Necessary Energy For Prolonged Cardiovascular Workout.

5. Incorporate Flexibility Activities Like Yoga Or Pilates Into Your Workout Regimen. Engaging In These Activities Can Enhance Flexibility, Lower The Likelihood Of Injury, And Promote General Health.

6. Ensure Adequate Hydration, Particularly As Plant-Based Diets Are Often High In Fiber, Necessitating Water For Appropriate Digestion. Hydrate Before, During, And After Physical Activity.

7. Prior To Working Out, Eat A Well-Rounded Lunch or Snack. This May Involve A Combination Of Carbs And Plant-Based Proteins To Supply Energy And Aid Muscular Function.

8.   Post-Workout   Nutrition:
Replenish Your Body With A Post-Exercise Meal Or Snack Containing A Combination Of Carbohydrates And Proteins. This Facilitates Muscle Repair And Restores Glycogen Reserves.

9. Plant-Based Protein Sources:

• Make Sure To Obtain Sufficient Protein From Plant-Based Sources Such As Legumes, Tofu, Tempeh, Nuts, Seeds, And Whole Grains. Consider Using Protein Supplements If Necessary.

Consistency Is Crucial, And Engaging In Activities You Find Enjoyable Can Help You Maintain Dedication To Your

Fitness Regimen. Regardless Of Your Food Preferences, Integrating A Balanced Diet With Consistent Physical Activity Is A Potent Method To Enhance Your General Health And Wellness.

Conclusion

Ultimately, Embracing And Upholding A Vegetarian Lifestyle Offers Several Health Advantages And Ethical Reflections. An Organized Vegetarian Diet Can Supply All Essential Elements, Including Protein, From A Range Of Plant-Based Source. It Is Crucial To Prioritize A Varied And Well-Rounded Diet That Includes A Combination Of Fruits, Vegetables, Whole Grains, Legumes, Nuts, And Seeds.

• Maintaining A High-Protein Vegetarian Diet Requires Careful Meal Planning, Knowledge Of Nutritional Requirements, And Awareness Of Protein Complementarity.

Incorporating Protein-Rich Plant Foods, Using Plant-Based Protein Supplements As Needed, And Monitoring Overall Nutrient Consumption Are Essential For A Balanced And Nutritious Vegetarian Diet.

• Aside From Nutritional Decisions, Including Consistent Physical Activity Into A Vegetarian Way Of Living Can Improve Overall Health. Integrating Cardiovascular Exercises, Strength Training, And Flexibility Workouts Enhances Overall Fitness And Enhances The Health Advantages Of A Plant-Based Diet.

Success And Longevity In A Vegetarian Lifestyle Depend On Education,

Adaptability, And Personalized Strategies. Seeking Advice From Healthcare Professionals, Licensed Dietitians, And Fitness Experts Can Offer Tailored Recommendations According To Individual Health Objectives And Interests.

Adopting A Vegetarian Lifestyle Involves Not Just Eliminating Some Items From Your Diet But Also Including A Variety Of Nutritious Plant-Based Foods. By Carefully Planning And Dedicating Oneself To Holistic Health, People Can Flourish On A High-Protein Vegetarian Diet, Reaping The Advantages It Offers In Terms Of Personal Health,

Environmental Sustainability, And Ethical Concerns.

THE END